The Shocking Truth about Diseases that Cause Hair Loss

**Secrets You Need to Know About Losing Hair
So You Can Stop From Going Bald**

James Dobovin

Introduction:

I first started losing my hair when I was about 45 years old.

Of course, I panicked and started trying to cover the remaining hair with strange hairstyles that made me look silly in strong wind.

In compiling my hair information books my goal was to amass both informative and useful information.

Entwined in my words are long scientific words that are necessary if you decide to do further research. If they bother you just skip over them.

Along the way I found it difficult to locate facts about hair loss that was understandable and centrally located. Not wishing others to have such a difficult time I decided to put them all in one place. My individual hair information books include Male Hair Loss, Female Hair Loss, Saving Your Hair and Hair Diseases.

I sincerely hope that you learn some useful facts that will help you in your quest to save your hair.

Thanks and make it a healthy hair day.

James Dobovin

Disclaimer

It is sometimes found that a particular hair loss cause is more commonly related to a particular hair disease. In this context one can refer to the acquired hair shaft defects. These defects are usually triggered by the excessive use of hair treatments and styling products.

Hair diseases and hair loss are interrelated. One cannot be thought about without the other.

Common hair loss causes:

No single factor can be marked out as the universal cause of hair diseases. There are several causes varying from person to person.

The two types of hair loss diseases.

The hair loss causes can be broadly divided into the following two groups

The temporary effect and the one involving a prolonged action, usually triggered by genetics.

a.)The temporary effect – Usually such cases can be cured by medications and treatments.
b.)Prolonged hair loss diseases – Such cases may require long term treatment. Sometimes the drug treatment might appear to be ineffective. In such circumstances surgery like hair transplantation may be the way.

The causes of temporary hair loss include the ones like child birth, using birth control pills, etc.

Another key factor can be hormonal imbalance. It can have a severe impact by causing pattern baldness. The latter comes in the list of major hair diseases.

Relation between hair diseases and hair loss

It is sometimes found that a particular hair loss cause is more commonly related to a particular hair disease. In this context one can refer to the acquired hair shaft defects. These defects are usually triggered by the excessive use of hair treatments and styling products.

Similarly, infectious diseases have their root in unhygienic scalp.

The common causes of hair loss diseases include the following –

- Hormonal imbalance
- Ailment
- Faulty hair styling
- Inadequate diet

Hormonal Imbalance

In men – Hormonal imbalance is a major cause of hair loss diseases among men. The male hormone testosterone plays a key role in actuating hair loss. The enzyme 5 alpha reductase in the hair follicles turns testosterone into dihydrotestosterone (DHT). The latter is the most potent androgen promoting male pattern baldness, the common hair loss disease.

In women – Imbalance in thyroid hormone is a key cause of sudden hair loss among women. The thyroid gland's being in the state of overactive and under active might cause hair to fall.

Thyroid hormones largely influence cellular metabolism of scalp proteins, carbohydrates, lipids and minerals. And the hair matrix cells are highly affected by the thyroid hormones' excess or deficiency.

Hormonal imbalance also causes hair loss during pregnancy. Pregnancy witnesses a high level of estrogen hormones. This causes hair follicles percentage in anagen growth phase. But post-child birth there is a rapid fall in the estrogen level. Consequently a large number of hair follicles shift to a catagen phase. And gradually hair falls.

Women may also experience hair loss during post-pregnancy period. It is generally temporary in nature. But if it continues for months, then it may indicate hormonal imbalance in the body. And hormonal imbalance for an extended period requires proper treatment.

Ailment

Some of the serous ailments like high fever, severe infection, or flu may lead hair follicles to a resting phase. This condition called telogen effluvium results increased hair fall. But it is a temporary condition soon to be followed by normalcy.

Some cancer treatments also prevent the hair fiber growth. The hair becomes thin and breaks off. And gradually hair loss occurs. The condition starts within one to three weeks after the beginning of the chemotherapy treatment. The treatment may witness the patients losing up to 90 percent of their scalp hair.

Faulty Hair Styling

It means using certain hair styling techniques resulting in hair loss diseases like traction alopecia. In this condition the hair fibers are pulled out from the hair follicle by a hairstyle that pulls on the roots of the hair fibers. One example of such faulty hair styling is braiding cornrowing.

Cosmetic treatments like bleaching, coloring or hair straightening like chemical relaxing can also create problems if proper procedure is not followed.

Inadequate Diet

Taking up crash diets for rapid weight loss may lead to hair loss. Such diets are low in protein, vitamins and minerals, thus causing malnutrition. Abnormal eating habits lacking important nutrients can also result into hair loss.

Andropause and Hair Loss

Andropause and hair loss go together. Imagine clumps of hair falling off your head, or observing strands of once healthy hair collecting in the shower drain. Maybe you run your hand through your hair and feel it thinning. It can feel daunting and quite scary.

Typically, hair loss is a result of an imbalance of male testosterone hormone in the body. Instead of infusing the hair with healthy testosterone, enzymes break it down to a simpler form known as dihydrotestosterone.

An excess of this hormone has the effect of decreasing the size of hair follicles which eventually break down and make your hair fall off sporadically. The medical condition that is best associated with hair loss in Andropause sufferers is hyperthyroidism.

Hyperthyroidism is a by-product of decreasing levels of Human Growth Hormone, which is responsible for regulating our aging process.

Andropause sufferers' hormones have a profound effect on the rate and consistency of hair loss. Dihydrotestosterone (considered by medical circles the strongest, most potent form of testosterone) is responsible for building and growing body hair in men (at normal levels - an excess causes hair degeneration.)

This includes body hair, pubic hair, head hair, armpit hair – any hair. DHT is directly produced in the skin, made to work by supporting enzymes that break it down for distribution throughout the body.

DHT levels are present more in certain areas of the body than in others – explaining why we may have a full crop of hair on our heads and little bushes of hair on our chests and backs. Women also have DHT in their bodies but produce less of it.

That explains why women don't have body hair. Case in point: an excess of DHT is prevalent in Andropause sufferers, explaining the reason for hair loss. The enzyme used to break down testosterone to dihydrotestosterone is ¨over activated¨ - working too hard and too fast.

This is the primary cause for this Andropausal condition. As mentioned earlier, dihydrotestosterone is present more in certain areas of the body than in others. For this reason, men's hair can fall into funny patterns.

The balding train station clerk you might have seen with more hair on his scalp than the top of his head. The shrinking of hair follicles as a result of the production of DHT is attributed to this.

How hair grows is a wondrous thing in itself that needs to be recognized. Typically, hair grows at a rate of a quarter inch every 2 weeks. Andropause sufferers have their ¨hair growth cycles¨ disrupted when there is erratic growth of some hair strands where ¨new¨ hair pushed ¨old¨ hair out.

Because Andropause is a period of hormonal imbalance, a lack of hormonal stability and poor homeostasis (holistic balance) in the body pushes things out of whack.

If you want to maintain healthy strands of hair, one thing you can do is hit that stair climber machine! Exercise reverses the aging process and may certainly reverse this symptom. There are also hair loss products that can help you recapture your hair.

Secondary cause of hair loss in men suffering from Andropause is stress.

More specifically, stress raises the levels of cortisol and cortisone (known as stress hormones) in the body. Eating non-nutritional foods also speeds up hair loss.

Pretty much any activity that speeds up the aging process will speed up your hair loss.

Stay away from caffeinated drinks, fast foods, and cigarette smoking to keep running your hands through your thick mane longer. Participate in recreational activities to reduce stress and light up your life with a proper exercise regimen.

If you're suffering from this condition, don't let it affect you in the least bit!

Andropause should not serve as a punishment – rather, a realization of a future for the better.

Cause of Trichotillomania

Trichotillomania is a psychiatric condition in which an individual has an uncontrollable urge to pull out his or her own body hair. It is rather a compulsive behavior, in which the person finds very hard to stop the urge to pull body hair. It is believed that genetics is a cause of trichotillomania. The compulsive behavior like trichotillomania can sometimes run in families.

The term "trichotillomania" comes from the Greek words "thrix," meaning "hair" and "tillein" meaning "to pull" and "mania," the Greek word for "madness" or "frenzy". As the name suggests trichotillomania is a psychiatric condition in which an individual has an uncontrollable urge to pull out his or her own body hair.

For people suffering from trichotillomania, hair pulling is more than a habit. It is rather a compulsive behavior, which the person finds very hard to stop. The cause of tricholomania is supposed to be the imbalance of chemicals in the human brain.

People with trichotillomania pull their hair out of the root from places like the scalp, eyebrows, eyelashes, or even the pubic area. Some people even pull handfuls of hair, which can leave bald patches on the scalp or eyebrows. Other people pull out their hair one strand at a time.

Some inspect the strands after pulling them out or play with the hair after it's been pulled. About half of people with this condition also have the habit of putting the plucked hair in mouth.

Trichotillomania has been mentioned as a disorder in very early historical records. But clinically the condition trichotillomania was first described in 1889 by the French physician Francois Hallopeau. The condition is rare - statistics show it affects only 1% to 3% of the population, although new research suggests that the rate of hair pulling may be around 10% or higher.

Trichotillomania affects about twice as many girls as boys. Most people who have trichotillomania develop the condition during adolescence. However, it can start when a person is as young as 1 year old.

Trichotillomania is often the cause for embarrassment, frustration, shame, or depression for those people affected with the disorder. Those people also suffer from low self-esteem.

They usually try to hide their behavior from others. Because of this fact, social alienation is common in trichotillomania patients. Moreover, the patients also try to cover patches of balding scalp by wearing wigs, hats, scarves or hair clips, or by applying make-up or even by tattooing.

Doctors don't know much about the cause of trichotillomania. It is believed that genetics plays a major role. The compulsive behavior like trichotillomania can sometimes run in families.

Some psychiatrists think it might be related to OCD since OCD and trichotillomania are both anxiety disorders. This is one reason why the impulses that lead to hair pulling can be stronger when a person is stressed out or worried.

Experts think that the actual cause of tricholomania is the imbalance of chemicals in the brain. These chemicals, called neurotransmitters are part of the brain's communication center.

When something interferes with how neurotransmitters work it can cause problems like compulsive behaviors.

Since trichotillomania is a medical condition, it's not something most people can just stop doing when they feel like it. People with trichotillomania usually need help from medical experts before they can stop.
With the right help, though, most people overcome their hair-pulling urges. This help may involve therapy, medication, or a combination of both.

There are therapies in which special behavior techniques are used to help people recognize the urge to pull hair before the urge becomes too strong to resist. The patient learns ways to resist the urge so that the urge becomes weaker and then goes away.

Many people find it helpful to keep their hands busy with a different activity (like squeezing a stress ball or drawing) during times when the urge of pulling hair is strong. Even activities like knitting while watching TV seems to help.

Causes of Folliculitis

Folliculitis results from the infection of the hair follicles. Along with the inflammation the infectious pustules also result in hair loss. Bacteria, fungi, virus and parasites are folliculitis causes which are responsible for infection to the follicles from where it may spread to the other parts of the body.

A follicle refers to a crust or cavity from which the hair emerges on the surface of the skin. The term folliculitis is used to describe the inflamed condition of the hair. Depending upon the causal organism, folliculitis causes can be characterized as follows:

- **Bacterial Folliculitis**
- **Fungal Folliculitis**
- **Viral Folliculitis**
- **Parasitic Folliculitis**

Bacterial Folliculitis

Bacterial folliculitis develops when bacteria enters the body through a cut, scrape, surgical incision, or multiplies in the skin near a hair follicle. The bacteria can get trapped and the infection may spread from the hair follicles to the other parts of the body.

Bacterial folliculitis may be superficial or deep. Superficial folliculitis, also called impetigo, consists of pustules which are small-circumscribed elevations of the skin containing pus. The pustules are often surrounded by a ring of redness.

Deep folliculitis results when the infection goes deeper and involves more follicles to produce furuncles and carbuncles. These are more serious than folliculitis and can cause permanent damage and scarring to the skin.

Bacterial folliculitis usually occurs in children and adults. Staphylococcus aureus is the most common of bacterial folliculitis causes. It also causes sycosis, a deep chronic infection that involves the entire hair follicle.

Besides the species of streptococcus, pseudomonas, proteus and coliform bacteria have also been indicated as of bacterial folliculitis causes. "Hot Tub" Folliculitis is a condition caused by the pathogen pseudomonas aeruginosa.

This disease is often caused due to unsanitary conditions at a spa. The pathogens identified in Gram-negative folliculitis include Klebsiella, Enterobacter, and Proteus species. This type of folliculitis sometimes develops in people receiving long-term antibiotic treatment for acne.

Some superficial follicle infections spontaneously resolve themselves. However, bacterial infections like impetigo, furuncles, carbuncles and "hot tub" folliculitis may not resolve spontaneously and generally require prescription therapy.

All these infections are typically diagnosed by clinical presentation, after which predisposing factors are identified and eliminated.

Fungal Folliculitis

As the name suggests fungal folliculitis is caused due to fungal infections. Superficial fungal infections are found in the top layers of the skin; deep fungal infections invade deeper layers of the skin.

The infection from hair follicles can also spread to blood or internal organs.

The dermatophytic fungus, pityrosporum fungus and the yeast candida folliculitis are the prominent among the fungal folliculitis causes.

Dermatophytic folliculitis is caused most often by a zoophilic species, i.e. fungal species that show attraction to or affinity for animals. The condition presents as follicular pustules around a hardened erythematous (reddened) plaque. A deep fungal penetration causes a high degree of inflammation and determines the extent of hair shaft loss that occurs due to the infection.

Tinea capitis or ringworm of the head is the most important form of pediatric dermatophytic folliculitis. The clinical features of tinea capitis vary considerably depending on the species responsible for the infection. Typically, there is partial alopecia with a varying amount of inflammation.

In the non-inflammatory variants, asymmetrical lesions with short broken hair, 1 to 3 mm in length, are observed. Slight inflammation with scaling may be observed on careful inspection.

The most severe inflammatory reactions are called kerion and produce painful boggy masses studded with pustules. These lesions can result in severe hair loss and significant scarring when the disease is in advanced stages.

The diagnosis of tinea capitis is established by identifying the organism in infected hairs under the microscope. A diagnosis is often confirmed by cultures.

Tinea barbae is a superficial dermatophytic infection that is limited to the bearded areas of the face and neck and occurs almost exclusively in older adolescent and adult males.

The clinical presentation of tinea barbae includes deep folliculitis, red inflammatory papules and pustules with exudation, crusting and associated hair shaft loss. The two main species causing the infection are T. mentagrophytes and T. verrucosum.

Pityrosporum folliculitis is caused by pityrosporum yeasts resulting in an itchy eruption. The lesions are reddish follicular papules and pustules located mainly on the upper back, shoulders and chest. Candida folliculitis is caused by the Candida species, ubiquitous fungi that most commonly affect humans.

Viral Folliculitis

Viral folliculitis involves a variety of viral infections of the hair follicle. Infection by the herpes simple virus (HSV) often progress to form pustular or ulcerated lesions, and eventually a crust.

Infection caused by molluscum contagiosum indicates an immuneosuppressed state which manifests as multiple whitish, itchy papules over the beard area. There are also some reports of folliculitis caused by herpes zoster infection.

Parasitic Folliculitis

Parasites causing folliculitis are usually small pathogens that burrow into the hair follicle to live there or lay their eggs. Mites such as demodex folliculorum and demodex brevis are natural hosts of the human pilo-sebaceous follicle.

Hair Loss: Don't Rule Out a Thyroid Condition

If you suffer from hair loss you might want to make sure that your problem is not caused by a thyroid condition. Although the usual reasons for hair loss are genetic predetermination, hormonal changes, or certain cancer treatments, thyroid hair loss should also be considered.

There are three types of hair loss; thyroid hair loss, autoimmune alopecia, and male pattern hair loss. Thyroid hair loss can manifest in both hyperthyroidism and hypothyroidism. In those with thyroid hair loss, there will be a general thinning of the hair, without the bald patches characteristic of male pattern baldness.

Symptoms of hypothyroidism include fatigue, dry skin, abnormal sensitivity to cold, constipation and depression. If you one or more of these symptoms along with loss of hair, think about getting tested for thyroid problems.

Synthroid is commonly prescribed in hypothyroidism; this medication is effective however, it can produce thyroid hair loss as a side effect for some people. Your hair loss may be due to Synthroid, so speak to your doctor about the possibility.

Thyroid hair loss can also occur if you are under-treated. A Thyroid Stimulating Hormone level of around 1-2 is optimal for a large number of people who are suffering from hypothyroidism with no hair falling.

Evening primrose oil supplements are one alternative therapy that some have found to be useful in alleviating thyroid hair loss. Aromatherapy is another which is reported to be effective.

Essential oils of thyme, cedar wood oil, lavender, and rosemary can be blended and applied to the scalp to help encourage hair growth.

Ayurveda medicines such as Bhingaraj oil or brahmi oil have also been used to treat hair loss due to thyroid conditions. Both these oils applied to the scalp continuously for at least 3 months are said to aid hair growth. Growth of hair will also be aided by supplementation with the ayurvedic herbs amla and ashwagandha.

The ultimate remedy for thyroid hair loss is hair transplantation. Tiny hair plugs are removed from the scalp's back or side and then implanted to bald portions of the scalp.

Results can be seen after several months. This procedure is expensive and is not always covered by insurance providers, but can be worth every penny for those suffering from this discouraging condition.

Hair Loss- Are You Suffering From Alopecia Aerata?

Hair loss is a common problem. But most of the people who suffer hair loss never understand why their hair is falling. It is a mystery for most of us. Because of not understanding, we try many therapies including different diets and natural formulations. But most of the times, we find no improvement.

That is very disappointing and we accept the fact of hair loss and stop trying. This need not be done. Once we understand all the possible reasons of hair loss, we can surely find out what is happening to us and take an informed decision. Alopecia aerata is one of common causes of hair loss. Let us find out about that.

Hair loss- what is alopecia aerata?

Alopecia aerata is an autoimmune disease. In this disease the body attacks the hair follicles and kills them. The body begins to think that hair follicles are foreign objects and wants to remove them. Why it does that is a mystery.

Hair loss pattern in alopecia aerata

You may begin losing hair in coin size patches. Sometimes the loss will stop after a patch or two and re-grow there after some months. Sometimes the loss continues and you may lose all the hair.

This hair may come back after some months. No body can predict about how you will lose hair and when you will get it again.

If you have a family member who suffers from a autoimmune disease such as Atopic dermatitis, hay fever etc. your probability of getting alopecia aerata increases. There is no way to stop this hair loss. Only treatment can be done to get the hair back sooner.

Hair Loss Caused By Lichen Planus

Lichen planus is more of a skin disorder that also affects other areas of the body. Thus, it can not only affect the skin and body, but also the scalp. When the scalp is affected, hair loss is experienced.

There are several factors that can result in hair loss. One common disease is a disorder known as lichen planus. This particular disease is not in itself a direct cause but it is an important trigger and often causes complications with the scalp and can lead to this problem.

Lichen planus is more of a skin disorder that also affects other areas of the body. Thus, it can not only affect the skin and body, but also the scalp. When the scalp is affected, hair loss is experienced.

Licen phanus is usually considered to be an allergic reaction and is often associated with a poor immune system. Some believe that lichen planus is triggered from excessive stress.

Stress weakens the body's immune system and render it susceptible to infection and other health symptoms such as hair loss. The chances of getting another lichen planus attack rise with the first affliction, even with treatment and prevention measures.

Lichen planus is most identifiable by the changes in the skin that occur. There will be itching in certain areas of the skin, as well as skin lesions that will appear in a variety of places. The skin lesions will have a variety of attributes related to their shape, size and color, all which will help you in identifying the disorder.

There may also be nail abnormalities, such as ridges in the nails that begin to appear. The skin lesions will then begin to move into the mouth area and cause your mouth to feel dry. From here, lichen planus will begin to show on the scalp area and hair will be lost from the irritation from the scalp area.

Once you notice these symptoms, do not wait too long to treat the lichen planus. In most cases, the symptoms are not severe enough and will simply go away over time. However, there is also the possibility of the symptoms become full blown and it will be more difficult to treat at that point in time.

For treatment, you can take prescribed medications. Antihistamines are useful in helping to treat lichen planus. Vitamin A in the form of ointments and creams are also considered to be effective.

It can be expected that this disorder will disappear after a few months or after a longer amount of time. Also, ensure a healthy diet and lifestyle to boost your immune system.

If you notice both the above mentioned symptoms and also experience hair loss at the same time, then it is possible that you can be having lichen planus. To be absolutely sure, it is best to seek a professional diagnosis.

Lichen planus can cause much discomfort to you as it affects your physical appearance. Understanding what the symptoms of lichen planus are and knowing what to do will help you repair your skin and treat yourself from hair loss.

Hair Loss Scalp Disorder: Seborrheic Dermatitis

There can be several disorders or diseases that result in hair loss. Hair loss is an indication that there can be a problem that is happening inside your body. One disorder that is related to the changes on the scalp is known as seborrheic dermatitis. This is a common inherited disorder and should be treated continuously and as soon as possible.

Seborrheic dermatitis is also often known as dandruff, eczema or cradle cap. When you have seborrheic dermatitis, you experience a change in the skin texture on your scalp. This will include either greasy or oily areas over the scalp or white flakes that are coming from your scalp. You are also likely to experience itching and redness in the scalp area, and also hair loss.

If you notice any of the above mentioned symptoms, then you may be having seborrheic dermatitis. For treatment, you can use a medicated shampoo for direct application on your scalp. Depending on the shampoo, it will contain a variety of ingredients that will help.

If the medicated shampoo fails to arrest your hair loss and scalp disorder, you can get a prescribed medication from a health care provider in order to get rid of seborrheic dermatitis. These shampoos will contain medications such as salicylic acid, coal tar, zinc, resorcin and selenium.

The prescribed medications will have stronger amounts of these ingredients in them, as well as added ketoconazole and corticosteroids. You can also massage your head in order to get the balance in the scalp back to a normal condition. This is especially effective with children who are dealing with seborrheic dermatitis.

While seborrheic dermatitis can easily be treated with the right shampoos and care for the hair, it cannot easily be prevented. Once you have the symptoms, it will be likely that you may get them again. You will need to continue to use the shampoos that have the medication in them and take the necessary measures in order to prevent the problem from coming back.

In addition, make sure that you have an adequate supply of essential vitamins and supplements. As always, a healthy diet helps. Adopt good hair care tips to prevent more hair loss.

If you are having a difficult time from preventing this problem, then you can consult a health care provider about possible treatments. Having an understanding seborrheic dermatitis and knowing how to treat the problem will help you in maintaining a healthy scalp and hair.

How to Treat & Cure Alopecia

An article about how to treat and cure Alopecia to stop thinning hair and baldness

My Uncle has been a sufferer from the condition alopecia for many years. Like all sufferers of alopecia we search for how to treat alopecia and its cures in the hope that soon we can return back to a full head of hair.

Only recently he won the battle so I decided here to write about how he treated alopecia and the cures that actually work for other people with alopecia.

Thinning hair had dramatic effects on me personally. The feelings of anxiety are common when alopecia starts. As a previous sufferer of alopecia all i did was worry about my thinning hair when all i wanted to do was just live a normal life.

The pressures of society to look beautiful projected in glossy magazines and media advertising only go to make matters worse for the sufferer with sometimes feelings of isolation taking effect. The psychological factors of anyone losing their hair at any age can be catastrophic.

It has been estimated that 50% of men aged up to 50 years old suffer from alopecia and 40% of woman suffer from alopecia by menopause age.

1.7% of the population overall, including more than 4.7 million people in the USA alone suffer from alopecia and most don't know how to treat alopecia. A figure of close to a million people has recently been suggested for the United Kingdom population alone and as we can see it's a lot more common than we think.

Over 25% of people around the world who are affected by alopecia usually have someone within their family who have or had to treat alopecia at some stage of their lives.

Some studies have shown a link with between alopecia and stress or trauma of some kind.

In male and female pattern baldness, the culprit is something called dihydrotestosterone, or DHT, which is derived from androgen which is a male hormone. Circulating through the bloodstream, androgen is converted to DHT.

Those with greater enzyme activity have more DHT binding to their hair-follicle receptors. If flooded by DHT, the follicles sprout thinner hairs during the the normal recycle period until eventually nothing regrows.

Treating alopecia can take months if not years. If you start now and incorporate a routine into your daily lifestyle, before you know it the alopecia will be gone.

Why Plugged Hair Follicles Thin Your Hair and What You Can Do

There are many reasons why your hair thins or you become bald. One reason is your hair follicles become plugged. Discover in this article how you can un-plug your hair follicles so that you can stop hair thinning and perhaps grow more hair.

Losing your hair to where it thins or you become bald does not have to happen. Just by understanding why your hair falls out and thins allows you to take counter measures. Discover what counter measures you need to take to keep your hair full, thick, or from thinning.

There are various ways to keep your hair clean, shiny, and thick. If you still have hair and want to keep it or if your hair is starting to thin out, here are some hair remedies that you can use.

When your hair starts to thin down, three of the reasons are:

1. Your hair follicles are slowly becoming plug and preventing hair from growing out

2. Your hair is not receiving the nutrients it needs to grow and stay strong

3. Your hair is not getting enough blood circulating in your scalp

Plugged Hair Follicles

Just like acne, your hair follicles can become plugged. In acne a plug follicle results in sebum and bacteria becoming trapped in the follicle, which leads to an infection known as a pimple.

When a hair follicle becomes plugged on your scalp, the hair in that follicle becomes trapped and is prevented from coming to the surface. Over time, your scalp becomes smooth and you become bald or lose most of your hair.

So the secret to preventing hair loss, thinning and balding is to prevent your hair follicles from becoming plugged. Once you know what causes your follicle to plug, you can avoid or counteract those conditions.

Here is what causes your follicles to become plugged:

1. Excessive build up of testosterone in blood converting over to DHT and plugging up your hair follicles

2. Use of shampoos, conditioners, and gels that contain excessive un-natural chemical that stay on your scalp and get trapped in your follicles

3. Excessive release of sebum and scalp flaking mixing together to form a hard material that plugs up your follicles.

DHT Build Up in Your Follicle

It is well known now that excessive conversion of testosterone into DHT accumulates in the hair follicles and plugs. Knowing this you can use a variety of shampoos on your hair to dissolve this DHT. This keeps your pores open and your hair growing normally. You can also take capsules that prevent the conversion of testosterone into DHT.

Un-natural Shampoo and Conditioners

Most shampoos, conditioners, and hair gels are created using petrochemicals, un-natural additives, dyes, preservatives that are harmful to your hair and scalp.

In addition, these un-natural hair product chemicals get into your pores and can plug. Once in the follicle, they also get into your blood and are harmful to your liver and the rest of your body.

Search for more natural shampoo products which contain fewer petrochemicals and have more herbs with natural cleansing chemicals

Some people have oily hair and some dry. When the hair follicle releases excess sebum it accumulates on the scalp. Here it will combine with dirt, dead scalp cells, and shampoo chemical residues.

Using natural remedies reduces the amount of chemical available to combine with excess sebum and dead scalp cells. If you use any type of gel to style your hair these gels combine with sebum to plug up your follicles.

To keep your hair and scalp clean and follicles open, use aloe vera gel mixed with a few drops of jojoba oil. Buy aloe vera gel, 99% pure and pure jojoba oil. Put some aloe vera gel in your hand and add 4-5 drops of jojoba oil. Rub your hands together then rub this mixture into your hair. This mixture will keep your hair shiny and thick and your hair follicles open.

Just making these changes to your hair care will go a long way in keeping your hair from thinning any further

www.ingramcontent.com/pod-product-compliance
Lightning Source LLC
Chambersburg PA
CBHW080832310526
45788CB00019B/3315